# Outsmart the Common Cold

## The Quest to Never Get a Cold Again

*Steve Mueller*

First published in 2016

OUTSMART THE COMMON COLD

First Edition

Disclaimer:

This book is presented solely for educational and entertainment purposes. The author and publisher are not offering it as health or other professional services advice. While best efforts have been used in preparing this book, the author and publisher make no representations or warranties of any kind and assume no liabilities of any kind with respect to the accuracy or completeness of the contents and specifically disclaim any implied warranties of merchantability or fitness of use for a particular purpose. Neither the author nor the publisher shall be held liable or responsible to any person or entity with respect to any loss or incidental or consequential damages caused, or alleged to have been caused, directly or indirectly, by the information or programs contained herein. Every human is different and the advice and strategies contained herein may not be suitable for your situation. You should seek the services and advice of a professional before beginning to put any content of this book to practice.

The information provided in this book is designed to provide helpful information on the subjects discussed. It is sold with the understanding that the publisher is not engaged to render any type of psychological, medical legal, or any other kind of professional advice. Neither the publisher nor the author shall be liable for any physical, psychological, emotional, financial, or commercial damages, including, but not limited to, special, incidental, consequential or other damages. Our views and rights are the same: You are responsible for your own choices, actions, and results. This book is not meant to be used, nor should it be used, to diagnose or treat any medical condition. For diagnosis or treatment of any medical problem, consult a physician. The publisher and author are

To those who are tired of the common cold.

# Contents

# The Purpose of This Book

*"Man cannot discover new oceans unless he has the courage to lose sight of the shore."*

**André Gide**

For more than 15 years, I posed myself one question over and over again: "Why do some people never have a common cold?" It was the very question that always began to emerge whenever I was coming down with the common cold. Every single time an infection made me feel terrible and exhausted, I wondered how these individuals could make the seemingly impossible possible. Annoyed by my suffering, I simply could not help but feel great envy towards those who apparently have "superhuman" abilities when it comes to fending off common cold viruses.

Whenever I was feeling miserable as a result of a common cold infection, I wondered what a life without the common cold would be like. The more I suffered, the more I began dreaming of a life without having a runny nose in the most embarrassing situations. My fever-induced daydreams sparked the vision of a life in which one does not wake up with a painfully sore throat that makes it almost impossible to speak. In short, I figured living a life that is not continuously interrupted with common cold infections would be much more worthwhile. Even more so, I concluded that if the common cold were not a part of my life, many aspects of it would be much easier.

The problem, however, was that I never really believed it was possible to escape the common cold. During wintertime, I had one cold infection after another–just like everyone around me–without even considering that there could be ways to prevent such infections. Back then, it was simply much easier for me to regard the tiny minority that never came down with a cold as incredibly lucky individuals. This, in turn, proved to be quite a limiting mindset. If these people's "ability" to avoid common cold infections is reduced to sheer luck, it means that their results are not reproducible.

It was this kind of thinking that proved to be a major obstacle for me. Instead of actively seeking for potential solutions, my attempts to reduce the incidence of cold infections were halfhearted and–consequently–not at all fruitful. I was fairly convinced that there is no way to escape the common cold, which is why I neglected the subject for many years. Surely,

I made some superficial experiments with vitamin C, regular exercise, and healthy nutrition. But as anyone can tell you, these things are not that particularly effective when it comes to preventing common cold infections. These ineffective attempts even further convinced me that there was no escape from the common cold.

If it hadn't been for all the discomfort that came along with cold infections, I would have readily accepted my fate. But the more I suffered, the more determined I became to do something about it. This kind of insistence was quite a challenge in itself, especially during the initial stages of my quest. On the one hand, I was firm about affecting change. On the other hand, I thought it was impossible to do so.

Understandably, I felt trapped. Back then, it seemed to me as if there's no way to prevent the common cold. Over and over again, I asked myself if a high level of determination was enough to fight an enemy that seemingly could not be defeated. It was during this stage that I struggled the most. Was I wasting my time by trying to do what is considered to be impossible?

Nobody that I contacted during this challenging phase was of any help, either. From physicians to scientists, nobody considered it to be possible to avoid common cold infections. It seemed to me as if they all had accepted the common cold as something that could not be prevented. Admittedly, I fully agreed with them at that time.

My own experiences had shown me time and time again that it was not possible to prevent the common cold. But there was one thing that kept me going: the knowledge that there are people who never catch a cold infection. Whenever I asked an expert about the reasons why some people never come down with a common cold, I was looking into confused faces. No one seemed to have an answer to my question. Or rather, no one could give me a satisfying answer. Some even attributed these people's extraordinary gift to sheer luck. It was the cluelessness of the experts that motivated me to keep going. The answers I received from scientifically trained professionals and experts in the field were nothing but dissatisfying. However, I don't blame them for not knowing an answer to my question. Quite the contrary, it slowly began to dawn on me that there was possibly no way to answer my question.

At this stage of my quest, I was just as clueless as the experts. Despite this, I was quite thankful for their lack of potential explanations. It showed me that not much research was being conducted in this area, which is why getting answers from the scientific community would prove to be difficult.

My discussions with the experts made me aware of the fact that research in this area was stagnating. Common cold infections were simply accepted as a given by large parts of the scientific community, which is why the research focused on potential remedies to alleviate the symptoms. This approach is quite logical but also a little too uncritical in my opinion.

During this time, I noticed that there existed a large number of (online) articles in renowned (online) newspapers and scientific journals, stating confidently that there is no way to cure a common cold. I read every single article I could find but was quite disappointed at the lack of critical thinking in these publications. While many authors–especially journalists–were pretty assertive in convincing their readership that nothing could be done to cure an ongoing infection, the question if colds could be prevented was entirely omitted. What slightly irritated me was the fact that most journalists simply equated "no way to cure a cold" with "no way to prevent a cold." The underlying message of most publications was pretty straightforward: "There is no way to cure the common cold, don't bother wasting your time."

While I agreed with the authors that the common cold could not be cured, I felt as if the big elephant in the room was entirely ignored. Why was nobody addressing the fact that numerous individuals have managed to stay cold-free for years?

At this point, I understood that I had to explore the subject matter on my own if I ever wanted to make progress. This kind of self-initiated exploration made it necessary to conduct my own experiments in order to generate valuable insights. The results of my experiments, in turn, would allow me to gain an understanding of the factors that may potentially be of help in preventing common cold infections.

My willingness to experiment on my own marked an important shift in focus. Instead of focusing on the opinions of the experts in the field, I began investigating those who actually managed to stay cold-free for years. I figured that these individuals would be far more helpful in finding answers to my questions than experts who had preconceived opinions about the subject matter. The words "preconceived opinions" are not at all meant to be insulting. They are simply derived from the understanding that experts who have an average of 3 to 4 cold infections each year may be biased to a certain degree.

The great difficulty, however, was to find individuals who had not had a single cold infection for years. As we all know, these individuals are quite scarce. In fact, there's not a single person in my entire social circle that is part of this exclusive club. But once I did unearth some of these individuals and investigated their behaviors, I became even further discouraged. For many of them, being cold-free is the most natural thing and nothing they had to struggle for. Some are even as perplexed about the millions of people that are regularly coming down with a common cold as I was perplexed about their ability to stay cold-free. To make things worse, those who attributed their astonishing immunity to certain factors puzzled me even further. In fact, they all named a different factor as the reason for their astonishing immunity. Unfortunately, there was no common consensus amongst the members of the "cold-free club" about a particular remedy. Only much later I would begin to see the commonalities between many seemingly unrelated factors.

Once more, I was standing in front of a huge obstacle that assertively discouraged me from continuing my quest. Even those who remained cold-free for years couldn't exactly pinpoint the underlying reasons for their impressive immunity. However, turning around was not an option so I kept going. It was at this time that I decided to become a human guinea pig. If all the members of the "cold-free club" named a different reason for their immunity, I had to validate their claims on my own. Step-by-step, I began experimenting with those approaches that sounded the most reasonable and promising to me. My decision allowed me to gain important insights about what was working and what wasn't. Even more so, I began to discover the underlying commonalities between approaches that did not at all seem to be connected with each other. All of this helped me to refine my knowledge about fighting the common cold. Certainly, there were some days during which I made great progress. Unfortunately, there were many other days when yet another cold infection showed me in a harsh way that whatever I was working on at the time was not effective. But whenever I was confronted with these challenges, I always reminded myself of those individuals who had managed to stay cold-free for years. These individuals spurred my motivation and kept me going.

Today, I am one of them. But contrary to many of those who have been naturally cold-free for the greatest part of their lives, I had to work for it. Even though this was quite difficult at times, it allowed me to discover what works for regular people who are not gifted with levels of immunity that are above average. In fact, I became someone I was always looking to find during my research: someone who struggled greatly with the common cold for decades but somehow found a way to effectively prevent it.

Originally, I never intended to write my insights down. I was quite excited about seeing cold-free months turn into years, which showed me that I had finally overcome the common cold. At the same time, however, I felt quite powerless when it came to sharing my knowledge. Quickly I noticed that showing others that there are in fact ways to prevent the common cold was not that easy. Certainly, there were those who wondered why I was seemingly the only one who was never affected by a spreading cold virus. However, as soon as I began sharing my insights (I carefully omitted the most perplexing ones), people did not believe me a single word. To them, I was simply someone with a lot of luck and an even stronger immune system. Some even thought I was intentionally making fun of them. Not a single one did consider for a moment that I could be someone who has been working hard towards this aim for years. Unfortunately, I also noticed that it was far easier for them to ridicule my approaches than to actually test their validity. These experiences led me to conclude that writing about what I had discovered would not be greatly rewarding.

Knowing that my insights would be heavily criticized as soon as they are published, I delayed writing them down. At the same time, however, I was convinced that a great number of people could potentially benefit from what I had learned. In the end, I realized that if I could help one single person to live a better (and especially cold-free) life, it would be quite worthwhile to write this book and to endure criticism from those without the willingness to verify the validity of my claims. The decision was made and I began writing down what I had learned.

As I began writing this book, I always kept those in mind who greatly struggle with the common cold. I wrote this book speaking directly to the ones who are tired of having common cold infections. While writing, I always sought to address the problems of this group of people, which were, in fact, the same problems I was facing for a long time as well. What resulted from my work is an exploration of the–often times unusual–approaches that have provided great results for me.

But I also desired to go one step further than just writing about my experiences. For this reason, I've included numerous references to scientific studies that confirm my findings or substantiate my claims. In fact, this book references more than 45 scientific studies and relevant articles.

However, scientific studies and confirmatory research findings are not enough to overcome the common cold. What it takes is the willingness to put the contents of this book into practice. Without the desire to verify the claims made in this book, no progress can be accomplished. For this reason, I wrote this book for all those who are actually willing to make a change in their lives. This book is for you and everyone else who is tired of coming down with the common cold. To all the ones who want to challenge the status quo and those who are not happy with how things are when it comes to the common cold. This book is a companion for all those who are not satisfied with the already existing answers, those who are tired of taking expensive but ineffective medicine that only treats the symptoms, not the causes, of common cold infections. Here's to all those who want to take it a step further.

It's been a great honor for me to share the insights that I gained during my quest. I hope that you enjoy reading this book just as much as I enjoyed writing it.

STEVE MUELLER

# CHAPTER ONE

# Introduction

*"The greatest wealth is health."*

**Virgil**

**D**id you know that there is no escape from the common cold, no matter where you go? Scientific research has shown that cold-causing viruses (so-called Rhinoviruses) can be encountered in all corners of the world[1]. You can catch a cold even in remote places such as the Amazon or the Kalihi Islands. Hiding from the common cold on a deserted island is (unfortunately) not an option.

## Cold viruses can survive for days

To make things worse, cold viruses can survive indoors–under the right conditions–for more than seven days[2]. The cold-causing microbes remain infectious during this entire interval, even though their ability to spread the disease starts to decrease after 24 hours. Still, this is one full day during which the risk of picking up the virus is relatively high. Once the germs come in contact with your skin, all it takes is you to rub your eyes, scratch your nose, or bite your nails and you have caught an infection.

Just imagine how many surfaces you come in contact with in public. These touchable surfaces range from door knobs, light switches, elevator buttons to toilet paper rolls. Basically, handling any object an infected person just touched is enough to spread the disease. However, the most common way the germs spread is through a simple handshake or when you breathe in small droplets of someone's sneeze or cough.

**Is it possible to avoid the germs?**

As a result of the very long infectiousness of viruses, it is nearly impossible to avoid cold-causing microbes. There is no working strategy that allows you to prevent coming in contact with droplets laden with cold and flu viruses. If you really wanted to reduce this particular risk, you would have to wash and sanitize your hands right after touching any possibly infectious object.

This is not only a pain but also entirely useless if you come closer than 6 feet to a sick person. This is exactly the distance that virus-containing droplets can travel through the air, as a recent study suggests[3]. As a consequence, a common suggestion is to keep people who are coming down with a cold at a distance. This advice may be well-intended but it is very impractical–as anyone who works with people can tell. To make things worse, someone can already spread the cold virus before actually developing symptoms. In fact, only 75% of adults who have a cold virus infection actually develop symptoms of a cold, as scientific research suggests[4]. This leaves 25% spreading the cold viruses without even realizing it. They have no symptoms but can still infect you, which makes it even more difficult to avoid coming down with a cold.

If one cannot avoid coming into contact with the viruses that cause an infection, it is necessary to find another solution to prevent colds and flu. The tricky part lies in finding methods that actually work.

**The statistics**

There are over 200 different viruses that can cause an infection with the common cold[5]. The most common virus is the rhinovirus, coming from the word "rhin," which is Greek for "nose." The infection is called common cold for a good reason: each year people suffer 1 billion colds in the United States alone[6]. Moreover, it is the most common illness in humans. On average adults have 2-3 colds each year. Recovery from the common cold takes an average of 7-10 days, sometimes more[7].

The economic consequences of the common cold are dramatic. In 2003, a study was conducted with the intent of calculating the economic burden of non-influenza respiratory tract infections (common colds) in the United States[8]. The scientific researchers came to the conclusion that the war against the common cold costs the economy roughly $40 billion per year. Major cost drivers are missing days at work, which accounted for a total of 196 million days (126 million days alone for parents who had to stay at home for their sick child). For a more detailed analysis of the different cost types see Table 1 at the end of this chapter.

The study further highlights that Americans spend on average $2.9 billion on over-the-counter drugs for symptom relief. Another $400 million are spent on prescription medicines. The researchers also found out that doctors prescribe antibiotics for cold sufferers, even though it is commonly known that antibiotics do not work on viral infections. Out of all the participants in the study group, more than one-third received a prescription for antibiotics when they went to see a doctor. The money spent on purposeless attempts to alleviate the symptoms of a cold with antibiotics accounts to more than $1.1 billion annually (for roughly 41 million prescriptions), the study suggests.

This alarming data raises the suspicion that some doctors are either completely ignorant of the fact that they are prescribing inappropriate medicine with no effect whatsoever. Or, it is done on purpose. Needless to say, it does not matter which one of the two alternatives is actually the case. In the end, it is always you who suffers the consequences. You are unnecessarily spending money on medicine you do not need. $26.83 on antibiotics alone, to be precise. Combine that with the amount you spend for over-the-counter drugs and you get a hefty fine for coming down with a cold, averaging from $50-$85 per infection.

If you follow the instructions outlined in this book closely, you will no longer have to spend anything for the treatment of colds and flu. What I'm going to outline in the following is a $1 solution that helps you to stop an ongoing infection right in its tracks. This particular method is incredibly effective at preventing the outbreak of a common cold once you are infected. The technique is also able to alleviate the symptoms of a cold or flu infection and can reduce the duration of these illnesses significantly if it is applied a little too late to prevent the outbreak in the first place.

This, however, is only a quick-fix solution. It can be made use of right at that uncomfortable moment when you notice that you are coming down with a cold. And in this particular situation, it can work great wonders as it can stop roughly 80% of all common cold infections right in their tracks. But unfortunately, this particular technique cannot prevent getting infected with the virus. It is remarkably effective at stopping the outbreak of a common cold but that is just it.

The goal of writing this book, however, was to develop a system that could help you to prevent getting infected with the common cold virus in the first place. For this reason, many other highly effective strategies have been included in this book as well. One method is even so effective that common cold infections can become a thing of your past–if you practice this particular technique diligently and consistently.

*"An intervention that would effectively prevent or treat the cold would have a huge clinical and economic impact, far greater than for chronic diseases that we hear about [...]."*
**A. Mark Fendrick**

The impact of colds on the U. S. economy in detail:

**Table 1**

| Expenditures | in $ billion |
|---|---:|
| **Direct expenditures** | **$17.0** |
| - Physician services | **$7.7** |
| - Treatment of complications | **$4.8** |
| - OTC medication | $2.9 |
| - Prescription medicines | **$0.4** |
| -        Unnecessary        antibiotic prescriptions | $1.1 |
| **Indirect expenditures** | **$22.5** |
| - Missed workdays (childcare) | **$14.5** |
| - Missed workdays (cold infection) | **$8.0** |
| Sum total | $39.5 |

Data source: Fendrick et al. (2003)

# CHAPTER TWO

# History of the Common Cold

*"Those who cannot remember the past, are condemned to repeat it."*

**George Santayana**

The history of the common cold is quite a remarkable one. It can be safely said that the viruses responsible for common cold infections have launched successful and long-lasting careers in the area of "Human Annoyance." To make things worse, it does not appear as if these viruses are considering early retirement. Instead, they are full of sap and enjoy their domination over the human race.

But how came this unpleasant illness into existence? In the following, we'll have a concise look at the history of the common cold in order to explore everything we need to know about the arch enemy addressed in this book.

Even though the common cold is quite unpleasant and irritating, it normally passes quickly without causing side-effects. For this reason, cold infections were more or less accepted as an annoying but inevitable aspect of life. Even more so, our forefathers understood that the common cold does usually not cause serious health issues. They also knew that not much could be done about the infection. This is the reason why common colds were largely ignored in the history of mankind. It's also important to mention that historical societies were confronted with devastating epidemics, plagues, and pests throughout the centuries. A common cold infection looks pretty insignificant in comparison to many of these horrific outbreaks of illnesses. Consequently, the common cold did not attract much attention throughout the ages.

Interestingly enough, the earliest traces of references to the common cold date back to ancient China and Egypt. For this reason, it cannot be said with certainty when exactly the common cold began to emerge. It could be possible that our prehistoric forefathers were struggling just as much as we do with the common cold. However, it is also possible that cold infections arose much later during times when humans began to settle in villages and began picking up agriculture.

Unfortunately, Paleopathologists[9] know little to nothing about the way our forefathers treated illnesses during the

Stone Age. Therefore, it can only be speculated if mankind's earliest ancestors were suffering from common cold infections as well. What can be said with certainty, however, is that as soon as human beings began to settle in larger communities, cold infections began to spread. As the earliest seeds of civilization date back to approximately 9000 years ago, it can be assumed that common cold infections were spreading much quicker from this point onwards.

In the 30$^{th}$ century BC, the pharmaceutical works known as Pen-ts'ao were written by the ancient Chinese Emperor Shennong. His writings could possibly be the earliest traces of written instructions to use medicine for the treatment of cold- and flu-like symptoms. Whether or not these instructions really detailed the treatment of common cold infections is not known.

However, what can be safely said is that the ancient Egyptians were confronted with common cold infections. Dating back to 1550 BC, the Egyptian medical papyrus, also known as Ebers Papyrus, was addressing the symptoms of common colds and potential remedies. Back then, it was believed that drinking the milk of a mother could effectively alleviate the symptoms of the common cold. The underlying reason why this approach may have been beneficial is addressed in chapter five. (Don't worry, though, you don't have to drink breast milk to prevent common cold infections).

Specific references to the common cold began to increase during the Greco-Roman period, beginning in 332 BC. Hippocrates, one of the most remarkable physicians of this era, was perhaps the first to refer to the infection as a "common cold." Based on the works of Hippocrates, the Roman physician Galen further expanded the knowledge about the common cold. Dating back to the first century AD, the works of Dioscorides already detail various important medications for the treatment of common cold symptoms. The important works of Hippocrates, Galen, and Dioscorides were further elaborated on by Arabic physicians and became central aspects of medieval Arabic medicine.

During the Middle Ages, health conditions worsened significantly in Europe. One reason for this was the fall of the Roman empire, which resulted in a loss of important hygiene practices. Another aspect that contributed to declining health conditions was the fact that medicine became more and more dominated by religion. Therefore, illnesses, such as the common cold, were widely regarded as God's punishment, which could only be alleviated by intense prayer. To make things worse, treating illnesses by using herbal remedies was considered to be witchcraft, which was punished severely.

During the 15th and 16th centuries, things were beginning to change for the better. New inventions such as the printing press led not only to the establishment of scientific communities but also made knowledge about medicine more easily accessible. It was during this time that many important books were written and printed, which further helped to make important advances in medicine. In the 18th century, physicians and scientists began to gradually distance themselves from many ideas the ancients held about illnesses. In particular, their research showed them that the source of the common cold was not to be found in the head, as previously assumed by ancient writers, such as Galen.

The 19th century marked a period in which theories began to emerge which assumed that cold temperatures and poor functioning of the human skin could be the cause of common cold infections. Therefore, research during this time was especially centered on the human skin as a potential origin for the common cold. As such, it was believed that the common cold is the body's reaction to great temperature changes or exposure to cold temperatures. In the second half of the 19th century, experiments slowly began to disprove these theories.

During the 20th century, speculations began to arise that considered viruses as the potential cause of the common cold. However, it took decades until these–often times heavily attacked–theories could be proven. In the year 1956, the speculations were finally put to an end by fragmenting the virus responsible for the common cold for the very first time.

## – CHAPTER THREE –

# Probing the Causes

*"The art of medicine consists in amusing the patient while nature affects the cure."*

**Voltaire**

As soon as the cold temperatures start to kick in, you will notice people coughing and sneezing everywhere you go. At first, this is nothing too unusual. It is not occurring very often, so you don't take much notice of it. But after some time has passed, you begin to realize that everyone around you is coming down with a cold. From the people you encounter in the public transportation system to your colleagues and family, everyone is sick. Runny noses and chesty coughs everywhere.

There's no getting away from it. One can take precautions, such as sanitizing one's hands, only to find oneself coming down with the common cold, again and again. It feels as if one is continuously exposed to a virus without having a chance of fighting it. Even more so, catching a cold seems like a grim lottery that randomly selects how many colds you will catch throughout the year. If there was only a way to opt out from it...

I had enough of it. I couldn't stand it anymore, which is why I decided to take a stand against it. This sounds like an incredibly stupid thing to do when keeping in mind that the common cold is regarded as an infection that cannot be cured. They say it needs to cure itself, which takes time. They also say there is no cure for the common cold or flu. I began to question my initial decision to stand up against the common cold before I had even started. Had I set my mind on something that was not possible? Would I just waste my time without accomplishing anything?

I tried to ignore these questions, but I couldn't. The only thing that kept me going during this stage was my desperation. I was desperately looking for any piece of information that would at least help me to reduce the incidences of common cold infections. I kept telling myself that if it was possible to achieve a significant reduction in the amount of colds, I could count myself a happy man.

At that time, I had no idea what a journey was lying ahead of me: a journey during which I felt like a human guinea pig. Out of desperation, I began to experiment with supposed remedies, even if I found them questionable. None of them seemed to work.

My initial failures were quite important. They helped me to develop an understanding of the remedies that did not work. Even more so, I began to accept the possibility of failure. As a result, my initial desperation started to decrease. My anger at this annoying viral infection started to fade away and was replaced by a deep and rational curiosity.

I began approaching things in a more rational manner, which led me to discover one important detail about the subject after another, many of which I had dismissed earlier. Instead of approaching the problem hastily without taking too much care of the important details, I began to structure my research. I read everything I could possibly read about the common cold. However, I was also keeping an open mind about unusual approaches that seemed to work for others.

The scientific papers I read were pretty blunt in telling me that there was no possibility of curing the common cold. Whenever I encountered a scientist stating this fact, my motivation decreased just a little more. But there was hope, something that fueled my ambitions. Even if the scientists were correct in their statements about the common cold, there was still one thing they could not explain.

None of them could explain why some people never catch a cold. Any scientist or doctor I asked was pretty confident that there was no cure for the common cold. However, their confidence began to tremble as soon as I began to inquire why some people seemed to be able to avoid colds entirely. Often times, I was looking into perplexed faces. Many said that these people were just maintaining a healthy nutrition combined with a lot of physical exercise and a very strong immune system. Others were more honest and told me that research into the habits of these people would be necessary if one hopes to find any relevant answers.

**Why some people never catch a cold**

I was not at all satisfied with the answers I got in my conversations. As I am a curious person, I began to investigate the reasons why some people never catch a cold. I was already amazed by the opinionated answers I had received, but I was not prepared to discover how clueless the rest of the scientific community was about this issue.

*"The most obvious reason [...] is simply that [they] are lucky."*
**Stephen Morse**, professor of epidemiology
Mailman School of Public Health at Columbia University[10]

Thanks, but no thanks. I really don't want to accept "luck" as a possible explanation why some people never get sick. That's a little bit too easy. If these people share certain commonalities, luck can most definitely be excluded from the list of potential reasons.

An explanation that is better, though not satisfying, centers on health, nutrition and poor behaviors. Based on this idea, people who suffer from chronic conditions, eat poorly, or engage in poor behaviors (smoking, drinking etc.) are more likely to catch an infection.

> *"Some people are simply healthier than others. There are people who lead healthier lifestyles [...] they are less likely to become ill and it is a milder illness."*
> **William Schaffner**, professor of medicine[111]
> Division of infectious diseases at Vanderbilt University school of medicine

This explanation sounds logical. However, it always leaves me wondering: there are so many people who lead an incredibly healthy lifestyle but still catch one infection after another. The same holds true for explanations which take into account regular physical exercise, plenty of sleep and proper stress management. Countless people do all these things but are still not able to prevent common cold infections.

Needless to say, I was not satisfied with these answers. In fact, it even increased my curiosity and spurred my motivation. I began to realize that even if the scientific standpoint was that one could not cure colds, some people seemed to be able to prevent it nonetheless.

In all honesty, preventing a common cold infection is even better than curing it, isn't it? If there is a way for you to prevent a cold, you don't need a cure. This important realization led to a major turn in my journey. Without this turning point, I would not have been willing to continue my journey. Luckily, I continued my pursuit, which led me to discover a remedy that is capable of preventing colds.

# CHAPTER FOUR

# Common Misconceptions

*"If a doctor treats your cold, it will go away in 14 days. If you leave it alone, it will go away in two weeks."*

**Gloria Silverstein**

Before we can develop an understanding of how to prevent an infection with the cold virus, it is important to outline false beliefs regarding colds and flu. This is an important step, as millions of people spend countless amounts of dollars in the hope of being able to prevent the common cold. However, as we all know too well, none of these supposed cures work. Let's have a look at the most common myths.

**Myth #1: Vitamin C prevents colds**

Contrary to the popular belief, vitamin C does neither help in preventing nor does it help in curing colds. In fact, its effectiveness is just as insignificant as the effect of a placebo.

Responsible for this misconception is the Nobel Prize winner Linus Pauling, who announced in his book entitled *Vitamin C and the Common Cold* that one could reduce the risk of a cold infection by 45% through the intake of 1,000 mg of vitamin C daily[12]. Pauling himself is reported to have taken a dose ranging from 12,000 mg to 40,000 mg daily. These amounts are not only 16 to 600 times higher than the RDA of 60 mg for vitamin C, it has also been proven to have no effect in the prevention of colds. To this date, more than 17 double-blind studies have been conducted to put the claims of Pauling to a test. None of them was able to support the claims he made. However, it was noted that such high doses were indeed able to reduce the symptoms of a cold slightly. One of the largest of these studies was conducted with 3,500 volunteers who received a daily dosage of 4,000 mg[13]. From such a huge data set, one can draw pretty good conclusions– in this case, that vitamin C does not prevent colds.

The megavitamin claims popularized by Pauling were clearly disputed countless times. However, an unsuspecting public accepted the claims, largely due to Pauling's prestige as a Nobel Prize winner. More than 30 years later, vitamin C is commonly regarded as a highly effective nutrient for preventing colds. Even more so, it is seen as an immune system strengthening vitamin. As a result, more and more people take costly vitamin C supplements in the hope that it helps them to prevent colds. Their hopes are in vain, as a study on vitamin C supplementation shows[14]. The research involving 11,350 participants showed that even if you take more than 0.2 g vitamin C daily, your risk of coming down with a cold does not decrease. The authors concluded:

> *"The failure of vitamin C supplementation to reduce the incidence of colds in the normal population indicates that routine mega-dose prophylaxis is not rationally justified for community use."*
> **Douglas R. M., et al.**[15]

Conclusion: vitamin C does not prevent colds and flu.

## Myth #2: OTC remedies cure colds and flu

Another very popular belief is that over-the-counter (OTC) medicine is able to cure colds. Nothing could be further from the truth! The most popular OTC cold medications come in the form of syrups containing alcohol, pain reliever, and antihistamines. One takes them after coming down with a cold, shortly before going to bed. They contribute to an excellent night's sleep, and in the best case you wake up feeling relieved and revitalized. At least, that's what clever marketers are trying to sell us.

While these kinds of over-the-counter medicines work to a certain degree in blocking and suppressing the symptoms of a cold, such as coughing, aches, fever, and congestion, they are not able to cure the infection. Instead, the cold infection remains. Your body is still infected. Only the symptoms of your infection are suppressed. This is a small difference, which has a huge impact. If you really want to prevent colds you have to get down to the root of the problem. Suppressing the symptoms of a problem can be counterproductive, especially in the case of common cold infections.

Conclusion: OTC remedies cannot cure colds.

## Myth #3: You'll only catch a cold when your immune system is weakened

If you ask random people on the street about what they think is important to prevent colds, they will always name two things. Firstly, they will tell you to take a lot of vitamin C. We already discussed this misconception in the above. Secondly, they will advise you to strengthen your immune system. The well-intended advice about increasing one's immunity is quite correct. A strong immune system can help to prevent some of the infections. What is not correct is that you will not catch a cold when your immune system is strong. To understand this point, it is necessary to elaborate. Generally, a weakened immune system is seen as a major factor that leads to a higher susceptibility to colds. After you have caught a cold and experience severe symptoms, you are inclined to think that your immune system is particularly weak at the moment.

This is a common misperception. Most people think that cold symptoms are the result of destructive cold viruses. What is actually the case is that cold symptoms are just the innate immune system's reaction to the viruses. If you are coming down with a terrible cold, it is a sign of a strong immune system, as it reacts strongly to the infection.

> *"[...] susceptibility to cold symptoms is not a sign of a weakened immune system, but quite the opposite. And if you're looking to quell those symptoms, strengthening your immune system may be counterproductive. It could aggravate the symptoms by amplifying the very inflammatory agents that cause them."*
> **Jennifer Ackerman**[16]

To answer the initial question, one does not only catch colds when the immune system is particularly low. This conclusion was drawn from a study, which exposed volunteers with cold viruses[17]. These volunteers were healthy adults. Yet, 95% became infected after exposure to the virus.

Conclusion: even with a strong immune system you can catch a cold.

## Myth #4: Exposure to cold causes common colds

Most people try to avoid cold temperatures as best as they can because they think becoming chilled can cause common colds. After all, most catch a cold during winter when it is cold outside. Drawing the conclusion that cold temperatures could be associated with a cold infection sounds plausible, right?

There exists one scientific study, which has looked at this particular question in detail[18]. Contrary to the popular belief, the research paper showed that infections with the common cold did not increase in the group of people who were chilled. Those who were exposed to cold temperatures did not develop more colds than the other group who were not chilled. The authors concluded:

> *"Thus, this study demonstrated no effect of exposure to cold on host resistance to rhinovirus infection and illness that could account for the commonly held belief that exposure to cold influences or causes common colds."*
>
> **Gordon Douglas, Jr. et al.**[19]

Despite the results of this study, cold weather might still have an impact on the number of cold infections, although an indirect one. It is known that cold and flu viruses are able to withstand cold temperatures[20]. The reason why flu infections start to increase during the winter season lies in the virus's response to cold temperatures. During warm temperatures the virus dries out and weakens, which makes it less infectious.

Quite the opposite is true during cold winter temperatures. When exposed to cold temperatures, the outer covering of the virus hardens. The protective covering of the virus melts upon entry into the body's respiratory tract. As a result, the virus is not dried out and remains highly infectious. Only in this state is the virus able to enter a cell and infect the body[21].

Conclusion: exposure to cold temperatures does not automatically lead to an infection with the common cold.

**Myth #5: Feed a cold, starve a fever**
"Feed a cold, starve a fever" might be the oldest myth in this list. Its earliest traces can be found in a 1553 dictionary by John Withals, where it is stated that "fasting is a great remedy of fever.[22]" The underlying idea behind this is that the body can generate more warmth through eating food, which was considered helpful when having a cold. The second principle behind this belief is that restraining from eating could assist the body in cooling down when overheated as a result of fever.

Even though the maxim is nearly 500 years old, it seems to have been handed down from generation to generation. However, thanks to the help of modern science it is now possible to evaluate the maxim's validity. The saying "feed a cold, starve a fever" is only partly correct. "Feed a cold, feed a fever" is correct.

But why is it helpful to feed a cold? When your body is under attack by an infection, it needs energy to fight the virus. This energy can be provided through food, as eating helps the body in generating heat. This effect, however, can also be achieved by keeping your body warm, for instance by staying in bed.

The reason why it is important to feed a fever, instead of starving it, is more intriguing. When you have an infection, the immune system responds by raising your body's temperature. In order to do this, it is necessary to increase metabolism, which is achieved through burning calories.

This process, however, requires a lot of energy, which is why it is important to take in calories.

Conclusion: feed a cold, feed a fever.

## Myth #6: After getting the flu you're safe for the rest of the season

Another popular belief is that after getting the flu, you become immune for the rest of the season. People believe that once you have an infection, you develop antibodies against the virus, helping you to avoid the same type of virus in the future. This, of course, is correct. But as we all know just too well, one can have several colds throughout the year. The same holds true for the flu.

The reason for this lies in the trickiness of the influenza virus. The dominant strains of the virus change continuously each year. Additionally, there are different types of the virus in circulation. So even if you have developed antibodies against one specific strain, it is still possible to be infected by another type of the virus.

The same applies to colds. It is even more likely to have several cold infections each year. The reason for this lies therein that more than 200 different common cold viruses exist. Even if you are immune to one type, it is very likely that you come in contact with another one that you are not immune to.

Conclusion: one can have several flu infections in one season.

## Myth #7: Antibiotics fight colds and flu

Many people assume antibiotics help in fighting a cold or flu. This topic was already addressed in the introduction of this book, but it is important to demystify this misperception once and for all: antibiotics cannot fight viruses.

Antibiotics are medications that support the body in fighting bacterial infections. Colds and flu, however, are caused by viruses. This means that antibiotics will have no effect whatsoever on colds and flu. In fact, antibiotics may do more harm than good, when taken during a virus infection. Taking antibiotics during such a situation may increase your risk of catching an infection that is resistant to antibiotics[23].

To make things worse, taking antibiotics when having a cold or flu can cause secondary bacterial infections (for instance pneumonia, ear infections, and bronchitis). This is a consequence of an immune system that is already weakened from fighting the cold or flu.

If your doctor prescribes you antibiotics when you're having a cold infection, breath in deeply, exhale calmly, get up slowly, and run as fast as you can.

Conclusion: antibiotics cannot treat colds and flu.


## Myth #8: A cold can turn into the flu

Responsible for infections with the flu or the common cold are two entirely different viruses. It is therefore not possible that a cold turns into the flu. If a person develops the flu, it originated from a flu infection in the first place. However, telling the difference between a common cold and the flu is challenging, especially during the early stages. The symptoms that come along with the flu are more intense than with a cold infection.

Conclusion: a cold cannot turn into the flu.

**Myth #9: If you have a cold, you need to sweat it out**
Trying to sweat out a cold is one of these desperate attempts that come with the frustration of not being able to cure a cold. The belief behind it is that the body can be assisted in fighting the virus by keeping it very warm. Sweating, however, will only help to a certain degree. Once infected, the body needs time to rid itself of the virus. This is a process which cannot be shortened through sweating.

Conclusion: one cannot sweat a cold out.

# CHAPTER FIVE

# The Breakthrough

*"The real voyage of discovery consists not in seeking new landscapes, but in having new eyes."*

**Marcel Proust**

Challenging problems often require unconventional approaches. Sometimes, it is not enough to address problems from the traditional perspective. If an issue cannot be solved with the traditional tools, one needs to find new aids that no one previously thought of. It's not enough to focus on that which is right in front of you. One needs to look left and right, but also up and below. No stone is allowed to be left uncovered if a solution has to be found.

The same holds true for our journey of discovering a remedy that helps to prevent the common cold. My willingness not to disregard unconventional approaches altogether helped me to discover the remedy that I am going to present you in the following.

In most cases, the unconventional approaches I did discover were entirely useless. I could disregard 99% of these supposed remedies as they were ludicrous. I couldn't believe my ears when someone told me that whiskey helps to cure a cold as the alcohol "burns them germs away [sic]." I was even more astonished when people advised me to drink a warm beer while taking a hot bath. As I said, most of these suggestions were well-intended but proved to be useless after (more or less close) examination.

There was one remedy, however, that was somehow different. Initially, I had dismissed it immediately due to its rather odd nature. I simply could not believe that it works. However, I did not feel comfortable by solely relying on my belief. What kept me looking further into this supposed remedy was my ambition to research any credible solution that would present itself during my research. I had no hope that this supposed solution would prove to be effective. Nonetheless, I started doing my proper research, hoping that I would quickly find the necessary evidence to disprove the claims made.

I hoped the research would be straightforward and easy. Yet, my hopes were in vain. I could not find the necessary evidence to file it as another ineffective remedy. Instead of being able to disprove the claims quickly, I had to read paper after paper, each leaving me more puzzled than before. Even though I was baffled, I continued. My interest in this remedy had been sparked. The more I researched and the more I learned about this substance, the more interested I became. Quickly, I began to realize that my initial dismissal of the remedy had been purely superficial and not based on the evidence.

Before I'm going to name this very interesting substance, I would like to show you the plain facts about this remedy.

**The facts**

Here are the key highlights (explanation and proper citation follows):

· It is a naturally occurring chemical compound, consisting only of water and oxygen

· Organisms produce it as a by-product of oxidative metabolism

· White blood cells produce this chemical compound to kill bacteria and fight infections

· FDA approved it as oral antiseptic agent

· High dosages of it can be found in the mother's first milk as it helps to boost the immune system of the newborn, which is why the ancient Egyptians advised people to drink it when suffering from a common cold infection

· Fruit and vegetables naturally produce the substance

· Cleans well water and drinking water, removes odors and iron from it

· Rainwater contains this substance naturally

Finally, after having presented the plain facts I can reveal the name of this remedy:

## Hydrogen Peroxide

Hydrogen peroxide is a naturally occurring chemical compound that organisms produce as a by-product of oxidative metabolism.[24] It can be found in every living material. White blood cells produce hydrogen peroxide to kill bacteria and fight infections.[25] In fact, research has shown that white blood cells depend upon hydrogen peroxide to detect wounds:

> *"The body uses hydrogen peroxide to sound the alarm when a tissue has been injured. As a direct result of this hydrogen-peroxide red alert, white blood cells come to the aid of the wounded site. [...] much to the researchers surprise, they found that hydrogen peroxide immediately appeared at the wound site, prior to the arrival of any white blood cell, and quickly disseminated into neighboring tissue."*
> **David Cameron**[26]

One study also stated:

*"This proved that the white blood cells 'needed' hydrogen peroxide to sense the wound, and move towards it."*

**Philipp Niethammer**[27]

In 1983, the US food and drug administration (FDA) approved hydrogen peroxide as an oral antiseptic agent. The products of **1.5-3%** grade hydrogen peroxide are classified in Category I, which means they are GRAS (generally recognized as safe) and effective.[28, 29] In 2003, it was stated by a Subcommittee of the FDA about the oral uses of hydrogen peroxide:

*"The Subcommittee concludes that hydrogen peroxide is safe at concentrations of up to 3 percent."*[30]

I already stated that hydrogen peroxide is a naturally occurring chemical compound. But what is really interesting about it is that it can be found in high dosages in the mother's first milk, which is called colostrum.[31] Apparently, it helps to boost the newborns immune system.

Furthermore, hydrogen peroxide is an important part of a number of drinking water disinfection treatment processes, as it is capable of removing iron and odors from water.[32] Not only this, research has also shown that hydrogen peroxide can be found in rainwater as well.[33] This is because the $H_2O$ in the atmosphere comes in contact with ozone ($O_3$), which creates $H_2O_2$ (hydrogen peroxide). As a result, the rainwater transports the hydrogen peroxide down to earth, where it is taken up by plants. It makes plants grow better and faster, which is why so many people recommend using rainwater instead of tap water for watering.

Hydrogen peroxide also kills disease organisms through oxidation. It offers, therefore, a wide variety of possible applications. For instance, your body produces hydrogen peroxide to fight infections, toxins, parasites, viruses, and bacteria. As a 3% grade solution, it is applied to treat sinus infections as a nasal spray but is also a popular wound cleaner. It can be used as an inexpensive but effective mouthwash that has anti-inflammatory properties. Thanks to its anti-viral, anti-fungal, and antibacterial characteristics, it serves as a treatment of toothache, if an infection is the root cause of the ache. Others make use of it as toothpaste by combining it with baking soda.

More interesting, however, is the use of hydrogen peroxide to prevent colds. Generally, it is commonly accepted that the rhinovirus (the virus behind the common cold) causes infections when it comes in contact with a human's eyes, nose, or mouth. One scientist, however, developed the hypothesis that cold and flu viruses infect the body through the ear canal. This theory was developed by Dr. Richard Simmons in 1928. It was largely ignored and faded into obscurity over the decades.

According to Dr. Simmons, the virus enters the inner-ear and begins to breed. From the inner-ear, the virus spreads and infects the body. Following along with this idea, an infection with the common cold could be treated by finding a remedy that could be applied to the location of infection within the inner-ear. This is where hydrogen peroxide comes into play. As a liquid solution, it can easily reach even the remotest areas within the ears.

Even though I was skeptical about the claim that cold and flu viruses infect the body through the ear, I kept researching. I considered an infection through the ear as one possible way of infection. As much as I was skeptical about Dr. Simmons's claim, I also found the "cold infection only through eyes, ears and mouth" statement of modern-day science questionable. Why could an infection not occur through all four channels?

I began to realize that the scientific theories would not be of any help. Instead, what I needed was practical experience of people who had already tested hydrogen peroxide as a potential cure for the common cold. I was able to find many testimonials, which only increased my interest in hydrogen peroxide. At first, I could not believe how many people had already made positive experiences with hydrogen peroxide as a cold remedy. The sheer amount of testimonies was just stunning.

I gave my best to read any review I could possibly get my hands on. It was a daunting task, but I considered it as tremendously important. Instead of only reading these reviews, I began to extract all the important information. I categorized the information in a separate spreadsheet and began analyzing it thoroughly.

Based on these reviews, it can be concluded that hydrogen peroxide seems to work outstandingly well. In fact, it was really difficult to find negative reviews. A large percentage of the testimonies were tremendously positive. More often than not I came across a person having a success rate of 100%. However, I also noticed that for some people the efficiency of hydrogen peroxide as a cold remedy was not 100%. Often, people reported that they were able to prevent a cold in 4 out of 5 times. This corresponds to a success rate of approximately 80%, which is still great. If you put these figures into practice, it means you can prevent 80 ongoing cold infections from 100. Or, to calculate it down for the time span of one year, you are able to cure 2.4 of 3 cold infections (assuming an average of 3 cold infections annually), which would nonetheless be fantastic.

One reason why some people have a lower success rate could be that they do not apply hydrogen peroxide as soon as the first symptoms of a cold appear. Many times I read reports of people who used the remedy days later. Yet, I was astonished to read that they reported, in many cases, a relief of symptoms. I was even more surprised to hear that they were able to reduce the duration of their illness. However, it is important to mention that hydrogen peroxide can only deliver its full benefits if it is applied immediately after noticing that you are infected.

The next chapter will address scientific studies that investigated the effectiveness of hydrogen peroxide. The chapter thereafter will show you precisely how to use hydrogen peroxide to prevent colds and the important details you need to keep in mind when using hydrogen peroxide.

# – CHAPTER SIX –

# Testimonies

*"What can be asserted without evidence can also be dismissed without evidence."*

**Christopher Hitchens**

I have included this chapter for one reason: I don't want you to believe me. I want you to be critical. I want you to question everything that I write. But I also want to give you an opportunity to investigate the claims made. Stating that one could prevent colds with a success rate ranging from 80% to 100% is pretty assertive. Normally, I prefer to use scientific sources to support my claims. However, when it comes to hydrogen peroxide we are facing an odd problem. There's not a single scientific study that has attempted to disprove the theory. Not a single one.

One really wonders why no such attempts were made, especially when thinking about the hundreds of people reporting success with the method. Usually, scientists are very quick in disputing any kinds of outrageous claims. This is not the case with hydrogen peroxide. There's no attempt to question hydrogen peroxide as a cold remedy. Instead, the topic is not even addressed. I am skeptical when scientists try to attack theories in an unscientific manner but I am even more skeptical when a theory with large amounts of evidence is entirely hushed up. Could one reason for this be that no scientist receives funding to investigate a potential remedy that costs $1? Potentially. If you have a look at the sponsors of scientific studies, you might be able to see a connection.

**Hydrogen peroxide (3%) can be applied to the ear canal** A common belief about hydrogen peroxide is that it is dangerous. This is partly correct, partly wrong. When we talk about hydrogen peroxide, we need to specify which concentration level of the solution we are talking about. When people think about hydrogen peroxide, they think about the (truly dangerous) hydrogen peroxide solutions that have a high concentration, for instance, the 30% grade type. These are the solutions used for bleaching and other purposes. The concentrated solutions are dangerous, indeed. They need to be handled with great care. One must never come in contact with this highly concentrated substance. However, the hydrogen peroxide that is used to prevent colds is diluted to 3%, meaning that it consists of 97% water and only of 3% hydrogen peroxide.

3% grade hydrogen peroxide is used, for instance, to remove earwax. One scientific study applied urea-hydrogen peroxide in the ears of the study participants and compared it to other earwax solvents.[34] In 1947 it was first discovered that hydrogen peroxide can remove earwax.[35] Scientists of the University of Virginia Health System discussed the use of hydrogen peroxide in the ear canal to remove earwax as well, stating that 3% hydrogen peroxide could be used to "fill [the] affected ear canal 15 to 30 minutes."[36] I could cite many other sources, but I hope you get my point that research about applying 3% hydrogen peroxide in the ear canal is conducted. None of them reported side effects if the 3% hydrogen peroxide solution was properly applied. The conclusion of these results is that hydrogen peroxide that is diluted to 3% can safely be administered into the ear canal.

How it was discovered that hydrogen peroxide could prevent colds, I don't know. I can only speculate that it was passed down as a home remedy from generation to generation, decades after the discovery of hydrogen peroxide in 1818. The remedy was popularized by Dr. Joseph Mercola, who conducted testing with patients of his clinic, reporting that many "have had remarkable results in curing colds and flu within 12 to 14 hours when administering a few drops of three percent hydrogen peroxide (H2O2) into each ear."[37]

When it comes to hydrogen peroxide as a remedy to prevent colds, there are two factions. The first group had the courage to test the effects of hydrogen peroxide and reported their own practical experiences with the remedy. The other group is very skeptical, stating that hydrogen peroxide is extremely dangerous (we already discussed this, 3% grade hydrogen peroxide is safe to use) or pointing out that it is useless, as colds and flu are transmitted through eyes, mouth, and nose. Not a single person of the second group tested the remedy. However, I was not able to detect an important third group: the group of people who put hydrogen peroxide to practice and had negative experiences with it or found it not helpful at all.

Therefore, I have chosen to let the reviews speak for themselves. Links to testimonies are included from a wide range of sources, to prevent bias.

One more thing I find necessary to mention is that I also considered the possibility that all of these testimonies are faked. I don't need to mention that this is nearly impossible when considering the vast size of reviews. I have also included testimonies of people with established accounts on forums that are not related to the subject at all. Some of them have 300 to 600 posts on these forums. These are no accounts that were quickly created to distribute spam. Furthermore, it is questionable if someone would create fake reviews for a $1 remedy that most households already have in store. But without further ado, here are links to the testimonies:

> *I heard many years ago that the cold/flu virus enters the body through the ears. As a healthcare professional, it seemed utterly ridiculous that anybody would be so "ignorant" as to believe this [...] I wasn't feeling well one day – actually, for about two or three days, and I decided – what the heck, I'll pour some peroxide in my ears, and see what happens. I swear, on all that is holy – I did this twice a day for two days, and when I woke the third morning, I felt SO much better! I don't know if the peroxide CURED me or not, but – my cold was gone – so, I don't care.*
> **Brian, OH, source:** Earthclinic.com

> *Everytime I feel a cold coming on, I put a drop of peroxide in my ears (for about 3-5 min. each), and by the next day I feel great.*
> **David, source:** CrossFit.com

> *I use food grade peroxide when I have colds or the flu. It knocks it out in less than 24 hours normally.*
> **Rivah, source:** Backwoodshome.com

**Author's note**: Some people speak of food grade hydrogen peroxide. Often times, this means that they buy the 30% food grade hydrogen peroxide solution and dilute it with water to 3%. They do this because it is sometimes difficult to find food grade hydrogen peroxide that is diluted to 3%. Never ever come into contact with the 30% hydrogen peroxide solution, this poses a terminal health risk, for instance when swallowed. As a general rule, you should never use hydrogen peroxide higher than the 3% solution.

*I tried it the last time I had symptoms of the onset of a cold. Works like a charm. [...] Initially I was also doubtful this would work. [...] and I thought hey why not give it a try. Nothing to lose. I recommend it to my friends now and they think I'm a quack.*
**Calvin, source:** Hardwarezone.com.sg

*[...] when I started feeling the symptoms of a cold come on, I decided to give it a shot. [...] you are supposed to use the peroxide as soon as you feel cold symptoms, but I waited until Monday night. Even then, it seems to have helped, since I am pretty much over the cold already, and the symptoms never really got that bad. [...] Usually my colds last about 10 days, but this one lasted 4.*
**Bigdummy, TX, source:** city-data.com

*I tried it a couple of weeks ago when I began to get a sore throat. [...] Over the course of the next few hours the sore throat went away. My 2 year old had a runny nose and began coughing which lasted for at least 4 days. [...] in this case we did not "catch" the illness at the beginning. However, I tried it anyway. [...] I expected him to get a fever again when the Ibuprofen wore off but the next day (Monday) he steadily made progress and this morning he is not sick! [...] I am SO GLAD that this "episode" was aborted and know that in the future, we will always use the H202 "cure" at the First Sign of an illness.*

**Agapemom, source:** curezone.org


*For the flu a couple of drops of hydrogen peroxide in each ear (this is where the flu starts) a few times a day is good.*

**J. Spade, CA, source:** bulletproofexec.com


*I have also tried the peroxide in my ears several times. I do think it shortened my cold considerably at least twice that I can pinpoint. With all the bubbling it sure \*sounds\* like something is being eradicated!*

**Heather, source:** Chriskresser.com


*My son was on antibiotics almost monthly for ear infections from 12 months to 2 1/2 years. [...] My chiropractor recommended hydrogen peroxide in the ear [...]. Last year my son woke up in the middle of the night screaming and holding his ear, I immediately assumed ear infection. All I had on hand was hydrogen peroxide so I put 1-2 drops in one ear, I think it tingled and he didn't like that so I followed it up with garlic oil. He was completely fine by the morning.*

**Jessica, source:** Kellythekitchenkop.com

# – CHAPTER SEVEN –

# Instructions

*"He who loves practice without theory is like the sailor who boards ship without a rudder and compass and never knows where he made cast."*

**Leonardo da Vinci**

Let's put what we have learned about hydrogen peroxide into practice. The following instructions shall help you to apply hydrogen peroxide in a safe manner. There are certain important aspects one needs to keep in mind when using hydrogen peroxide. They are all outlined in the following. Or, to turn the above-mentioned quote of Leonardo da Vinci around, theory is nothing without practice.

I have prepared a table which presents the key highlights, you can find it in the following. The key highlights are explained in more detail later.

**Use a 3% hydrogen peroxide solution to prevent colds**

Basically, hydrogen peroxide can be used to prevent colds, by administering 2-3 drops of 3% grade hydrogen peroxide into each ear.[38] The amount of hydrogen peroxide that is used depends, some administer 2-3 drops while others prefer to fill the ear canal entirety.

Table 2

| Key Highlight | Explanation |
|---|---|
| **Immediately** | Hydrogen peroxide needs to be administered as soon as the first symptoms of a cold/flu start to appear |
| **2-7 warmed drops** | Warm the H2O2 slightly before you apply it (to prevent ear pain) - warm tap water should be sufficient to increase the dropper's temperature (make sure that it is warm, not burning) |
| **3% concentration** | Only use 3% hydrogen peroxide; **Do not** use any hydrogen peroxide that is more concentrated than 3% (this is really important). |
| **Food grade** | Make sure that the 3% hydrogen peroxide solution is labeled "food grade", other solutions can contain |

| | |
|---|---|
| | contaminants |
| **5-10 minutes** | Administer it for 5-10 minutes in your ear canal; as a rule of thumb: when bubbling sound in your ear ceases you can drain it; leave it no longer than 10 minutes in your ear |
| **Switch ears** | Repeat this process with the other ear |
| **Repeat** | Should symptoms reside, repeat the whole process after 6-8 hours, at a maximum twice a day |
| **Avoid eye contact** | Avoid eye contact **at all costs**. No hydrogen peroxide should ever come in contact with your eyes; rinse eyes immediately with water if you get hydrogen peroxide in the eyes |
| **No daily usage** | Only use hydrogen peroxide when you have symptoms of a cold. You should not use it regularly or even daily. Also, do not use hydrogen peroxide when you're pregnant. |
| That's it. | |

Data source: healingdaily.com [39], mercola.com [40]

**Detailed instructions:**

It is important to administer the 3% hydrogen peroxide immediately after noticing the first symptoms of a cold/flu. These symptoms can range from scratchy throats, continuous sneezing, to runny noses. If the remedy is not immediately applied, it will loose its effectiveness to a certain degree. It can still be used, but it will not be able to prevent colds and flu. However, many people report that it also alleviates symptoms dramatically, leading to a significant reduction of the duration of their illness.

When using hydrogen peroxide, it is tremendously important to make sure that you use 3% hydrogen peroxide. Never use hydrogen peroxide that is more concentrated than 3%. If you come in direct contact with a 30% solution you are putting your health at risk. What some people do is that they buy 30% food grade hydrogen peroxide and dilute it down to 3%, by filling drops of the highly concentrated solution into water. If you do not know how to safely dilute 30% grade hydrogen peroxide, then, by all means, do not do it. Whatever you do, only administer 3% hydrogen peroxide. You should also make sure that the hydrogen peroxide that you use is labeled "food grade."

Some advice to warm the hydrogen peroxide slightly. (Applying cold hydrogen peroxide causes a slight stinging sensation in the ears). For this purpose, most put some of the hydrogen peroxide into a small dropper and allow it to warm up for a couple of minutes under warm tap water.

Before you administer the hydrogen peroxide, you can let one drop of it come in contact with the skin of your hand, in order to verify that the solution is indeed only concentrated at a level of 3%, as it says on the package. This is just a safety measure for your protection.

The best way to administer the 3% grade hydrogen peroxide is when you lie on your side. You can use an eyedropper for this purpose. Keep tissues ready. Make sure that the hydrogen peroxide does not get in contact with your eyes. You can use swim goggles to increase your safety. Should your eyes, however, come in contact with hydrogen peroxide, it is necessary to rinse your eyes immediately and to seek a healthcare professional.

Common sensations when administering 3% hydrogen peroxide into your ears are the hearing of bubbling sounds and you might feel a slight stinging or tickling. This is normal. A bubbling sound means that the hydrogen peroxide is fighting some kind of infection. If you administer hydrogen peroxide and you hear no bubbling sound, it means there is no infection.

Leave the hydrogen peroxide for 5-10 minutes in your ear, then let it drain into the tissue or sink. In general, you can let it drain as soon as the bubbling sound starts to cease. After this, repeat the whole process with the other ear.

Do not use hydrogen peroxide if you have no cold symptoms or when you're pregnant. Also, you should not use it regularly or even daily.

# CHAPTER EIGHT

# Continuing the Pursuit

*"Success is not final, failure is not fatal: it is the courage to continue that counts."*

**Winston Churchill**

**A**dmittedly, using hydrogen peroxide is a rather radical step to prevent the outbreak of a cold infection. Discovering its great potential was definitely an important milestone in my journey. However, it was just that–a milestone, not the destination. Seeing the amazing results of this remarkable remedy encouraged me to continue my investigations. While I was deeply satisfied with the results of my initial research, I definitely wanted more. On one hand, I was more than happy to finally have found a solution to my struggle with the common cold. On the other hand, I knew that it was only a quick-fix solution. Hydrogen peroxide works remarkably effective when it comes to fighting off a common cold infection, but if I had the choice, I would always prefer to prevent the infection in the first place. Consequently, despite my interesting discovery, in the back of my head there always remained the nagging feeling that hydrogen peroxide simply wasn't enough. Yes, it's effective but I prefer not having to use it, which can only be accomplished by discovering ways to prevent an infection.

I could have stopped at this point in my journey. A partial victory over the common cold was mine but I kept going. I wanted more. I constantly reminded myself that if there is one remedy with the potential to prevent a cold from breaking out, there must be others as well. The focus of my research began to change. Instead of experimenting with remedies that promised to alleviate or fight the symptoms of a cold infection, I sought to find solutions that would help me to prevent the entire infection instead.

In this sense, it was no longer a matter of finding something to treat an ongoing infection. It was now the quest to find methods and remedies that promised to maximize the chances of preventing the infection in the first place.

# – CHAPTER NINE –

# What's inside Matters

*"The road to health is paved with good intestines!"*

**Sherry A. Rogers**

As we all know, a healthy immune system can–to a certain degree–help us to prevent common cold infections. It is, therefore, only too understandable that most people advise you to boost your immune system when you ask them how you can prevent colds. Naturally, one way to do this is to integrate foods into your diet that allow you to support your immune system. But the more I investigated the immunity-boosting effects of certain foods, the more I began to see an underlying commonality. Many of these foods helped to improve the immune system by promoting a healthy gut flora. Interestingly enough, the individual cold-preventing effects of these foods were neglectable; what seemed to matter was their combined effect on the gut flora.

What many people, including my former self, seem to underestimate is the great impact our guts can have on our health. In fact, scientific research has highlighted time and time again that a healthy gut is critical to a person's overall health. At the same time, various studies have shown that unhealthy intestines are correlated with numerous diseases, such as chronic fatigue syndrome, diabetes, and arthritis. The reason for this lies in the fact that approximately 70-80% of your immune system resides in your gut. Hence, by improving your gut health, you can supercharge your immune system. Or, as Hippocrates stated more than 2000 years ago, "All disease begins in the gut."

If we really want to find an effective approach to preventing common cold infections, we definitely need to take our gut health into consideration. By improving the gut flora, or rather by restoring beneficial intestinal microbiota, we can promote overall health, as shown, for instance, in research published in 2003[41]. And once our gut health is improved, we are less susceptible to viral infections such as the common cold. Improving your gut flora, however, is not always that easy.

The number of microorganisms that can be found in your gut flora exceeds 1,000,000,000,000 (that is 1 trillion) by far. (Estimates range from 30-100 trillion microbes that can be found in the gastrointestinal tract). These organisms include bacteria, fungi, but also viruses. While many of these microorganisms have quite important functions, others are nothing but destructive. If there is an imbalance between the good and bad bacteria in your gut, a higher susceptibility to cold viruses is the likely result. Signs that your gut flora is imbalanced (i.e. that there are too many bad bacteria) include constipation, chronic diarrhea, excess intestinal gas, and chronic bad breath.

What is worse, your gut microbiota is under constant attack from external influences. These aggressors are toxins, antibiotics or chemicals that you ingest, for instance, through animal meat, polluted food, or agricultural products. Another risk comes in the form of the water you drink if there are chemicals added to it, in most cases this is chlorine.

Therefore, the first step in restoring the balance in your gut flora lies in avoiding those substances that wreck havoc on the microorganisms in your intestinal tract. Aside from the factors mentioned in the above, these negative influences also include sugar, refined oils, animal fats, and processed foods. Avoid these factors as best as you can, or at least limit consumption of these foods. Specifically, you should drastically reduce the amount of sugar you consume, including the sugar in fruit. It goes without saying that soft drinks, alcohol, antibiotics, and fast food should be avoided as well.

The second step consists of eating a diet that helps you to re-balance the microorganisms in your gut flora. Such a diet consists of whole foods that are rich in fiber like whole grains, seeds, nuts, beans, and vegetables. Changing your diet can already make a great difference. But in order to take it to the next level, you also need to ingest probiotics on a daily basis. These probiotics consist of good and beneficial microorganisms that will help you to improve your gut health while simultaneously reducing inflammation in the gastrointestinal tract. Interestingly enough, probiotics are not nourishing you, they are providing nutrition to the beneficial bacteria of your gut flora. By doing so, probiotics help you to keep the good microorganisms alive so you can benefit from their positive impact on the gut flora.

One fantastic source of probiotics can be found in traditionally fermented foods, such as sauerkraut (pickled cabbage) and kimchi. Other probiotic sources of beneficial bacteria include yogurt, kefir, miso soup, and natto. While probiotics do not seem to reduce the incidence of common cold infections, scientific research[42] shows that they can significantly shorten the duration of a cold. However, it's important to remember that this is the result of one study that only focused on two specific types of probiotic bacteria. There are much more with many different probiotic strains within every probiotic species. At the same time, there's a particular reason why probiotics alone cannot help you to prevent common cold infections, which will be discussed in the following. If the conducting scientists of the study had considered this factor as well, the research results could have turned out to be quite different.

As the above-mentioned scientific study highlights, probiotics alone may not be able to help us prevent an infection with the common cold. The reason for this is simple, probiotics help you in balancing your gut flora but they cannot help your gut to get rid of immune system weakening substances. In fact, these bad substances make it even more difficult to establish and maintain a healthy gut flora. One could eat huge amounts of probiotics, which is definitely not recommended, without long-lasting results–if one's intestines are loaded with toxic and harmful substances. Make no mistake, this is more often the case than most of us assume. Even people who eat healthily and do a lot of exercise are confronted with numerous pollutants day in and day out. The human body is not able to easily get rid of all of them, which leads to an accumulation over time. If we were now to assume that the mentioned scientific study was conducted with participants of average health, it is fairly safe to say that the effectiveness of the consumed probiotics was reduced by immune system weakening substances in the gastrointestinal tract.

In order to boost the immune system improving function of probiotics it is, therefore, important to remove toxins, heavy metals, and chemicals from your gut. Only by finding an effective way to accomplish this, a healthy gut flora can be established.

The intake of bentonite clay is a fantastic way to accomplish this. It promotes the reduction of unbeneficial bacteria so that beneficial microorganisms can be promoted. Bentonite clay accomplishes this by helping you in the removal of unwanted and havoc wrecking substances from the gut, such as toxins, heavy metals, and chemicals. The reason why bentonite clay is so effective at this is because it is a so-called "binder" that binds to unwanted substances and helps to excrete them. Among many others, bentonite clay binds to parasites, pesticides, pathogens, fungi, yeast, heavy metals, and bacteria. By doing so, bentonite clay cleanses the gut flora, which in turn boosts your immune system and makes you less susceptible to viruses and bacteria. And, it greatly boosts the positive impact of probiotics. If your gut is "clean," it is easier to maintain a healthy gut flora.

Due to the fact that bentonite clay is negatively charged, it effectively binds with most of the positively charged electrons that heavy metals, chemicals, and toxins consist of. Without this binding process, these negative substances could not be removed from your body. Again, this shows us why probiotics alone may not lead to the results we are looking for. Probiotics are microorganisms that become part of your gut flora. However, these microorganisms are not able to bind to negative substances in order to expel them from your body. As a positive side-effect, clay does also help you to maintain a strong gut wall. This is especially important because it prevents toxins, chemicals, and bacteria from entering the bloodstream, which helps you to live a healthier life. When there are no toxins and other substances that circulate in your bloodstream, your overall health will improve.

Interestingly enough, numerous traditional cultures have used the local type of clay available in order to protect themselves from disease. There are even records of indigenous cultures' use of clay dating back to prehistoric times thousands of years ago. Among Native Americans, bentonite clay is, for instance, called "the soil that heals." Indigenous people worldwide consider clay not only as an important healing substance but also an important detoxifier. In fact, it's an effective way to detoxify in a natural way. Aside from detoxification, clay is also a fantastic way to protect yourself from cold and flu viruses, as it binds to viruses and flushes them out of your system. Another important aspect of clay is that it stimulates certain actions in the human body simply by being present. This is called catalytic action, which can help in stimulating red blood cells (important for the immune system) and promotes better organ function.

Additionally, many important minerals, such as magnesium, copper, calcium, sodium, and iron, can be found in clay. It is, therefore, a natural source of essential minerals and vitamins. The minerals that can be found in clay are often alkalized, which helps to further alkalize your body. In doing so, it helps your body to balance its pH levels so that a healthy balance between alkalinity and acidity can be established.

Some even consider a body that is too acidic as one of the root causes for numerous health issues.

You can make use of all the beneficial effects of bentonite clay by ingesting it. In order to so, you can drink ½ up to 1 teaspoon of bentonite clay mixed in water. It's preferable to leave the clay for at least 30 minutes (several hours is better) in the water so that its positive electromagnetic charge is activated. It's always best to begin small and to slowly work yourself up. When it comes to clay, more is not necessarily better. You can think of clay as a powerful magnet. You don't necessarily need a huge magnet to get the job done. This will only overcomplicate matters. At the same time, it is important to remember that clay needs water to work its wonders. Otherwise, its drying qualities may make it impossible for you to ingest it. It is also important to mention that clay must never get in contact with metallic spoons or other objects that it can extract harmful substances from (a water glass is just fine). The ingestion of clay should be avoided when taking homeopathic or pharmaceutical medicine.

What is remarkable is that this approach manifested astonishing results when it comes to preventing the common cold. Roughly after three months of nutritional changes, eating probiotics, and using clay, the incidences when I resorted back to using hydrogen peroxide in order to prevent a cold infection from breaking out began to reduce. I was finally coming closer to my goal, which was finding ways to prevent the outbreak of common cold infections in the first place. My experiments further showed me what an important function the gut flora performs when it comes to immunity and the fighting off of infections. It was in this moment when I began to realize that certain methods to balance the gut flora and to rid it from unwanted substances could produce remarkable health effects not only restricted to the prevention of common cold infections.

The results of my investigation encouraged me to further explore the subject of detoxification. I also became quite interested in methods to get rid of parasites, especially in the gastrointestinal tract. These two methods are–to my present understanding–of the utmost importance to promote overall health. While especially detoxification practices do not seem to have the best reputation, they can improve one's overall health, if performed correctly, effectively, and most important of all: carefully. One particular study[43], for instance, highlighted that doing a relatively mild foot-supplemented detoxification program could already reduce the symptoms of chronic health problems by half.

However, as of writing this, my experiments with advanced detoxification programs had just begun, which is why I couldn't safely estimate whether or not they have an influence on a person's ability to prevent common cold infections. I think there is definitely a connection but this is merely an assumption–I prefer hard evidence as a result of experimenting for months. In my opinion, detoxification has a great potential but at the moment, I lack the necessary evidence that would justify an inclusion of such methods in this book. It's important to note that this does not mean that detoxification is not beneficial. It simply means that I haven't progressed far enough to safely come to the conclusion that detox can definitely contribute to the prevention of common cold infections.

The aforementioned lack of evidence is twofold. First of all, the techniques addressed so far have already helped me to reduce the incidence of common cold infections significantly. Second of all, at the time of writing this, my experiments with detoxification had not yet reached a stage where I could say that I have mastered it. For this reason, detoxification is not included in this book. It is, however, definitely a subject worth researching.

So far, the only results I can report stem from a rather aggressive approach of fighting parasites by using therapeutic grade garlic essential oil that is used in combination with cacao butter as suppository. Even though the results were absolutely astonishing, it is difficult to tell if they had an impact on the incidence of infections. I haven't had common cold symptoms for more than a year before beginning the "treatment," so the only conclusion I can come to is that it did not make things worse. However, the overall health benefits of the parasite elimination program were quite remarkable, especially when it comes to mental health, overall well-being, and energy level. This is the reason why I chose to shortly address this kind of treatment as well so that the reader may be in a position to choose for themselves whether or not they would like to further delve into this subject.

If you do explore this area, it's important to remember that using suppositories is always a lot more effective than simply ingesting certain substances. Suppositories help you to get a large portion of whatever substance you're using right into your bloodstream. This is so important because many substances that are ingested lose their potency long before they arrive at the intestines. In my parasite elimination experiment, I used therapeutic grade garlic essential oil and made ice cube shaped suppositories with it by using cacao butter. Alternatively, you can also use coconut butter and other therapeutic grade essential oils, such as the oils of onion, clove, wormwood, turmeric, and ginger. Especially when it comes to using essential oils, it is highly advisable, to begin with really small doses and to gradually work yourself up. At the height of my experiment, I was using around 55 drops per suppository and had pretty good results with one suppository per day.

# CHAPTER TEN

# The Holy Grail?

*"Our real discoveries come from chaos, from going to the place that looks wrong and stupid and foolish."*

**Chuck Palahniuk**

It took me a great deal of courage to include this chapter in the book you are reading now. Many long hours, I debated with myself whether or not I should include the following. In the end, I decided to let this chapter become a part of the book, as you can see. The results that are going to be addressed in the following are simply too powerful when it comes to preventing cold infections. Omitting what I had found was, therefore, not an option. I simply couldn't ignore the impact of the following method on my quest to prevent common cold infections.

The reason that made me reluctant to include this chapter is simple: what is going to be addressed in the following is plain out ludicrous. Yes, you read that right: the following is nonsensical, laughable, and unreasonable. The great problem is that even though the following technique sounds ridiculous and absurd, it provides remarkable results. The best results of this entire book. That's why I've included this chapter. I'd rather be ridiculed by a small minority who has not even tried the following tactic than excluding perhaps the most important piece of the puzzle from the sincere and open-minded reader. There will always be those who criticize and ridicule a given approach before even trying. But I am also aware that a large number of readers has the courage to give the following a try before forming an opinion about it.

Be advised that what is to come may sound rather weird and utterly absurd. What I ask is that you keep an open mind and even better: that you consider trying this method for yourself. The good thing about this technique is that it can be quite easily implemented in your life and that it is not at all radical or in any way dangerous. In fact, if you are not allergic to water, which I presume no one is, then you can safely apply the following. The only people that should not apply this technique are pregnant women, people with a history of schizophrenia or epilepsy, and people with a peacemaker. And yes, the following is not at all about taking cold showers but it also has to do with cold water, to be more specific: it has to do with ice.

In Traditional Chinese Medicine (TCM), it is believed that there is a pressure point in the body that can help us to promote overall health when stimulated. This particular pressure point is also known as the "Feng Fu point." Especially acupuncturists stimulate this pressure point because of its health-promoting effects on the entire body. It is located at the back of your head, to be more precise: at the base of your skull. The Feng Fu can be found right where the top of your neck connects to your skull cap. It is approximately at level height with the end of your earlobe, right at the hole-like spot where the neck ends and your skull begins.

The Feng Fu point can be stimulated by placing an ice cube (1x1 inch) on this pressure point for 15-20 minutes, twice daily. Doing it for at least 20 minutes is preferable. What is important, however, is to be consistent in the stimulation of the Feng Fu point, i.e. it needs to be done every day for at least three months. Those who give up earlier and those who do not practice diligently may not reap the benefits of this technique. It's absolutely no problem when you sometimes forget to practice. When you realize that you haven't practiced for a day or two, simply return to practicing twice daily. However, the gap between exercises should not exceed more than three days. I "practice" the Feng Fu technique after getting up and before going to bed on every day without exception because I've really come to love it. The more consistent you are, the better your results. Someone who only practices three times a week will never accomplish the same as those who practice twice daily.

Stimulating the Feng Fu point with an ice cube can be done while lying on your back or on your belly button (sitting is fine as well). Simply use a towel to hold the ice cube so that it does not melt from the heat of your fingers. The ice cube should only touch the area at the back of your head, not your fingers. Otherwise, it will melt too quickly. The easiest way, however, is to simply fixate the ice cube with a bandage at the right spot. What I do is that I simply wear an old cap that I don't mind getting wet. It helps me to keep the ice cube right where it needs to be while I'm busy doing more important things. In order to prevent cold water from running down my spine, I simply wrap a towel around my neck.

The first time you try the Feng Fu method may feel a little awkward, but you will quickly get used to it. The coldness of the ice cube may also be a little irritating in the beginning, but the cold sensation will disappear within one minute or so. After five or 10 minutes have passed, you might not even feel the ice cube any longer, even though it is still there.

The consistent stimulation of the Feng Fu point for more than three months can produce remarkable health benefits. While there are some benefits that can be noticed almost instantly, such as an alleviation of the symptoms of a headache, other benefits take a little longer to manifest. But once these benefits do emerge, they are quite impressive. However, it is important to mention that the Feng Fu method works in a rather subtle manner. There may be weeks where you don't notice anything spectacular. Simply be patient and continue practicing. If you feel a little euphoric while practicing (or shortly after), worry not, this is perfectly normal. Stimulating the Feng Fu releases endorphins, which is why you might feel a lot happier for no good reason.

Among many other things, stimulating the Feng Fu point with an ice cube is said to balance the autonomic nervous system. This may sound unspectacular at first, but an imbalance in the autonomic nervous system could be a major cause for health issues. The reason why balancing the autonomic nervous system is so beneficial is the fact that it controls almost all vital bodily functions. It controls your heart rate, digestion, and many more important functions such as breathing.

It is not too far-fetched to assume that an autonomic nervous system that is not functioning as it should, can cause great problems in the rest of the body. Stimulating the Feng Fu pressure point is also said to help in improving your cardiovascular system, the quality of your sleep, and the functioning of your digestive system. It further alleviates headaches and helps you to manage gastrointestinal disorders. It is also said that the stimulation of the Feng Fu point alleviates arthritis, joint pain, and hypertension. There are many other beneficial effects such as reductions in stress, depression, and fatigue. However, the most important result of stimulating the Feng Fu pressure point–at least in the context of this book–is that it eliminates common cold infections. If you consistently stimulate this pressure point for a longer period of time, coming down with a cold will one day become a long-forgotten aspect of your past.

What makes stimulating the Feng Fu point so effective is that it is not just a method that treats the symptoms of an illness. Instead, it influences a beneficial impact on the entire body by balancing and rejuvenating the autonomous nervous system so that the body can be brought back into a healthier physiological state. The simple act of stimulating this acupuncture point with an ice cube has, therefore, a great influence on the entire organism. After doing this for a certain while, first signs of healing will begin to emerge. This is often followed by a great improvement of overall health and well-being. As a result, it is quite possible that some diseases begin to slowly disappear or are at least alleviated. Another aspect that makes the Feng Fu "therapy" so wonderful is that it lifts your spirits, boosts your mood, and makes you feel a lot more energetic.

# CHAPTER ELEVEN

# An Effective Trio

*"There is something magical about three you know - a trio is tight and nicely economical."*

**Ian Williams**

In the previous chapters, I have presented you a way to prevent colds right at the onset. But let us assume you want more. Let us assume you also want to learn what you can do to further reduce your risk of an infection with the common cold. If you were able to do this, you would no longer have to rely on hydrogen peroxide to do the trick for you. Even though hydrogen peroxide is a quick-fix and works astonishingly efficient, it's even better when you don't have to use it.

In the following, I would like to present you a very effective trio that can help you to prevent colds. Before discovering hydrogen peroxide and the Feng Fu method, I have been using the following three remedies with great success. If I am not mistaken, I managed to avoid catching a cold for two years and one or two months. At that time, this was already a great success for me. Something I had never achieved before. However, it is important that these three remedies can only develop their full potential when they are combined. Using them alone makes them less effective.

**Ginger tea**

It has become a regular habit of mine to drink at least one cup of freshly made Ginger tea daily. Even though I have to admit that the taste is rather biting (it takes a little getting used to), I would not want to miss it. That is primary because of its positive benefits. When drinking a whole can full of Ginger tea, you will quickly notice comfortable warmth spreading throughout your whole body. The warming effect helps the body to sweat, which is seen as important to rid toxins, cleanse the lymphatic system, and to boost immunity.

In terms of fighting the common cold, Ginger has a very special property, as research suggests.[44] Scientists found that Ginger contains a chemical, which is especially effective at fighting the rhinovirus (the most common virus behind the common cold). This chemical is called "sesquiterpene" and has a high anti-rhinoviral activity, meaning that it aggressively fights the common cold virus.

Further research highlighted that ginger also has a positive effect on the immune system. In this research, the influence of ginger on an infection of the respiratory tract with the RS-virus (respiratory syncytial virus) was investigated.[45] The RSV infection has similar symptoms as the common cold, but can last longer. The aforementioned study found that viruses were prevented from penetrating human cells by the intake of ginger, which increased a person's chances of staying healthy.

The only thing you need to consider is that you should avoid ginger while you are pregnant/breast-feeding. People with blood disorders, gallstones, and hypertension should avoid it, too.

**Avoiding sugar**

Limiting your sugar intake to a slight minimum is a highly effective strategy to prevent colds. Yet, many people find it incredibly difficult to reduce their consumption of sugar. In fact, once you start investigating the subject, you will find that it is really difficult to avoid refined sugar. Refined sugar has become an ingredient in nearly everything that we eat and drink. It can be found in low amounts in the bread we eat and to very high dosages in the soft drinks we consume. Mind you, when I speak of sugar in this context, I mean refined sugars, such as table sugar and high-fructose corn syrup. This does not include the natural fructose that can be found in fruits.

The reason why it is so effective to prevent colds by avoiding sugar is complex and requires proper explanation. First of all, research has shown that eating sugar decreases the ability of white blood cells to respond towards bacteria significantly.[46] If you consume a lot of sugar, your body's defense system cannot respond effectively to bacterial infections. As a result, you get more easily infected. The scientists concluded that maintaining low blood glucose levels (through minimized consumption of sugar):

> *"[...] may provide a clinical method of enhancing the body's defenses against infection. [...] Thus, diet may play a key role in the resistance to infection."*
> **Albert Sanchez, et al.**[47]

Keep the aforementioned facts in mind, as they will relate to another side-effect of sugar: the consumption of sugar causes an increased inflammation in the body, as many studies have proven.[48] This fact alone is already pretty bad. But once we tie this information in with the decreased ability of the white blood cells to respond to bacteria, it gets really dire.

When inflammation occurs, white blood cells are the first-responders that fight the inflammation. We have learned that sugar causes increased inflammation in the body. As a result, the white blood cells have to respond to more inflammatory sites in the body. The more sugar you eat, the more centers of inflammation are created. This means that the white blood cells become so occupied in their task of fighting inflammation that they can no longer respond effectively towards infections. If the body's defense mechanism cannot respond properly to infections, you'll be experiencing more infections.

That was the scientific standpoint. If you really desire to prevent colds and flu in a natural way, it is a must to avoid sugar. It is definitely not easy to minimize one's sugar intake. Your body will crave for sugar for quite some time. This craving will start to decrease if you are persistent and stick to your decision. After a couple of months, there will be no more craving at all. By then, the body has grown used to eat no sugar. As a positive side effect, your blood sugar levels will no longer fall to the bottom, demanding for a quick increase in sugar intake.

**Taking cold showers**

We all know that taking cold showers is beneficial to the immune system. Nonetheless, no one seems to do it despite its positive effect. The reason for this is simple: if you have ever stood under an ice cold shower, you know the shocking sensation and how terrible it feels. It does not feel good at all. If you are not used to taking cold showers, it will feel extremely uncomfortable. And let's face it, a warm shower is much more pleasurable. However, on our mission to prevent colds naturally, taking cold showers is an excellent tool we have in our arsenal.

I have been facing the same situation as you do. I did not like cold showers at all. It just felt so uncomfortable and irritating. But after doing some extensive research about its positive benefits, I became so motivated and tried it out for myself. What I can report is that you will grow used to it after approximately 2 or 3 months. Taking a cold shower will always be a little irritating, but your ability to withstand the cold will increase quickly. After you have overcome the initial phase, you will find it a lot easier to take a cold shower. You might even start to appreciate its rejuvenating and refreshing side-effects.

But why are cold showers so effective when it comes to preventing colds? The sudden exposure to cold water causes the body to enter a fever that lasts for a couple of minutes. Through the heating process, the body is assisted in fighting bacteria and viruses. Furthermore, the immune system benefits highly from the short exposure to cold water. One study, for instance, has shown that brief immersion of the body by cold water caused white blood cells to increase significantly.[49] An increase in white blood cells is particularly beneficial as it contributes to increased immunity against bacteria and viruses.

Further research has shown that winter swimmers benefited from an increased anti-oxidative protection.[50] This is particularly helpful as it helps you in reducing the risk of disease. Not related to colds and flu, but still important, is the hypothesis that taking cold showers could potentially stimulate your anti-tumor immunity.[51]

**Increased effectiveness through combination**

This chapter has presented you three very effective tools that can help you to prevent colds (ginger, reduction of sugar intake, and cold showering). They all work from a different perspective but are very effective. However, they can only develop their true potential if they are combined. Individually, these remedies might be useful, but it is doubtful that they can prevent colds.

Using all three of them in combination, however, is tremendously effective. If you are willing to combine these three effective remedies, you will benefit the most. However, you need to take into consideration that there are no exceptions allowed. Persistence is key.

# CHAPTER TWELVE

# Further Remedies

*"If I knew I was going to live this long, I'd have taken better care of myself."*

**Mickey Mantle**

For those who can't get enough of effective remedies to prevent colds, I have included this chapter. It contains other remedies that are helpful.

**Liposomal Vitamin C**

There is a major problem with vitamin C: it cannot be absorbed properly by the body. If you take a moderate dose of 30-180 mg/day, 70-90% of the vitamin C is absorbed. However, the absorption rate decreases significantly when the intake amount is increased. At doses higher than 1 g/day, the absorption is less than 50%, leading to an increased excretion of vitamin C in the urine.[52]

Logically, if the body can only absorb less than 50%, one would simply take a higher dose of vitamin C. It is not that easy, however. If you take too high doses of vitamin C, it will have considerable side-effects, such as diarrhea and dental erosion.

So-called "liposomal" vitamin C could provide the solution. Basically, this type of vitamin C is called liposomal because it is encapsulated. Through this encapsulation, a compound is created that is more similar to cell walls than vitamin C alone. The similarity increases the absorption of the vitamin C through the cells. As a result, the bioavailability of the vitamin C increases drastically, without the negative side-effects.

A study investigated the differences between regular vitamin C and liposomal encapsulated vitamin C.[53] Interestingly enough, the higher effectiveness of liposomal vitamin C was supported by the research. It was proven that the bioavailability of liposomal vitamin C was approximately twice as high as the bioavailability of regular vitamin C.

> *"Here, we provide evidence that plasma levels following oral administration of liposomal ascorbate [vitamin C] can reach approximately twice the predicted maximum. These findings have previously unrealized implication for the use of oral vitamin C as a therapeutic agent for various diseases."*
> **Stephen Hickey, et al.**[54]

When we translate these results in light of our attempt to prevent colds and flu, an increased absorption of vitamin C could make an important impact. If higher doses of vitamin C resulted in an increase of white blood cells, the fighting of viruses and infections could be aided. However, liposomal vitamin C is a relatively new topic and further research is certainly required, especially on its ability to prevent (or alleviate the symptoms of) colds and flu.

## Brewer's yeast

Brewer's yeast is well-known, as it is used in the fermentation of beer. Its noteworthy health benefits are not so well-known. For one reason, Brewer's yeast is a probiotic containing important microorganisms and microbes. Through the intake of Brewer's yeast as a supplement, the digestive tract is aided in restoring the population of beneficial microorganisms. This can have a high impact on the body's immune system, as scientific research suggests. The results highlighted that the study participants who took Brewer's yeast had significantly fewer colds and flu than the placebo group. Furthermore, Brewer's yeast helped to reduce the duration of colds or flu.[55]

> *"Both incidence and duration of cold and flu-like symptoms were significantly reduced, including almost a full day of duration reduction [...]."*
> **Mark Moyad, et al.**[56]

If Brewer's yeast alone has the potential to decrease the possibility of coming down with a cold significantly, it could be even more effective if it is combined with the other remedies presented in this book.

# CHAPTER THIRTEEN

# Closing Words

This book has presented a wide array of potential remedies that help you in preventing colds. We have started our journey with one of the most effective "quick-fix solutions" for colds and flu, hydrogen peroxide. It is a tool that can be applied right at the onset of the first cold or flu symptoms. During this stage, hydrogen peroxide gives you a high chance of preventing the disease from breaking out. Hydrogen peroxide can be regarded as something that helps you at the last minute when you have no other options left. Should it, therefore, remain the only remedy in our arsenal?

The answer is no. While there are some who prefer to keep things simple by only using hydrogen peroxide to treat the symptoms of common cold infections, it is always preferable to find ways to prevent these infections in the first place. For this reason, the book continued in exploring other potential remedies to prevent common cold infections. The willingness to continue led us to another important discovery.

The second major insight of this book is presented with the Feng Fu method, which has the potential to stop common cold infections once and for all. If this ancient technique is applied consistently, it can balance the autonomic nervous system, which can improve a person's overall health.

One further step in preventing common cold infections lies in promoting a healthy gut flora and ridding the gut of unwanted substances such as toxins, heavy metals, and chemicals. To round things off, this book has also taken natural remedies into consideration. These highly effective remedies are there to prevent colds in a more natural way. If you make use of these remedies in combination with the three major techniques presented in this book, you will no longer depend on a potential cure for the common cold as the incidences of common cold infections will gradually reduce until you finally join the exclusive club of those who are cold-free.

However, it is important to realize that only by putting the materials of this book to practice, good results can be accomplished. This is especially true when comes to combining the various techniques outlined in this book. While individual methods to prevent common cold infections may be quite effective, a combination could potentially increase the body's ability to fight off cold viruses. As such, you will always get better results when you combine the various techniques presented in this book.

For starters, it can be quite helpful to start practicing the Feng Fu method and to gradually add further techniques, such as the strategies to establish a healthy balance in your gut, avoiding sugar, cold showering, drinking ginger tea, and eating Brewer's yeast.

Finally, it is important to note that even though hydrogen peroxide is astonishingly effective, it should always be considered as the last resort when you have no other options left. It would be unwise to stop at this point of the journey only because hydrogen peroxide does the job already pretty well. Instead, seek to become someone who does not only treat the symptoms of the problem but one who has learned to avoid the problem in the first place.

Last but not least, I'd like to wish you the best of luck in your endeavors.

# – CHAPTER FOURTEEN –
# Free Bonus Materials

This book was originally intended to be sold in a product package with various other helpful bonus materials for the reader. These additional products were designed to further help and assist the reader in the journey of becoming cold free. Unfortunately, it was not possible to bundle the book with its bonus materials on the marketplace it is sold (Amazon).

For this reason, it was decided to make the additional products freely available as bonus materials. These additional materials are available to all readers at no cost. It is my way of saying thank you for your support and the trust I received from all of you throughout the many years.

In the following, you can find an overview of these bonus materials and where you can download these products for free.

## 1. (Bonus) Prevent Cold Sores

Cold and flu infections go hand-in-hand with outbreaks of cold sores. These fever blisters are not only painful but also very embarrassing. What is worse, nothing seems to help in avoiding colds sores. There are (expensive) treatments but they only alleviate the pain or reduce the irritation. There are, however, some very interesting remedies that have the potential to prevent fever blisters right at the onset. These very special remedies are presented in this bonus product that accompanies Outsmart the Common Cold. It is a presentation that includes references to numerous testimonials of people who have applied these effective remedies with great success. At the same time, references to scientific studies that substantiate the claims made are included as well.

## 2. (Bonus) Superfoods That Prevent Colds

There are some very special superfoods that are astonishingly effective at boosting your immunity. These superfoods produce far better results than most other foods. However, the difficulty lies in knowing which foods to choose out of the list of numerous superfoods. This bonus product presents you the best superfoods that have the greatest impact on your immunity. Many of these foods will help you to ease the symptoms of ongoing common cold infections. But there are also superfoods featured in this presentation that could potentially help you to ward off infections in the first place.

## 3. (Bonus) Healthy Recipes

The body's immune system is constantly under attack. These negative side effects can be counterbalanced by a healthy nutrition. The cookbook presents you 10 healthy and easy recipes that help you to strengthen the immune system.

As promised, access to these bonus materials is freely available to all readers of Outsmart the Common Cold. All you need to do is send an email to service(at)planetofsuccess(dot)com with the subject line "Bonus Materials". [Replace "at" with an @-sign and "dot" with a "."]. Be sure to include, for instance, a screenshot of your product review on Amazon or any other proof that shows you've bought the book. Doing so helps us to ensure that the bonus materials are exclusively available for buyers of the book such as yourself. It is perfectly fine if you do not want to review the product on Amazon. The bonus materials come with no strings attached–all that is necessary is some kind of proof that your request is legitimate.

Feel free to get in touch with me if you need any further help.

# – CHAPTER FIFTEEN –

# Acknowledgments

**I** would like to make use of this opportunity to thank all the fabulous people who have supported and encouraged me throughout my journey. I am indebted to my parents, friends, guides, and teachers. Without you, writing this book would not have been possible.

I would also like to acknowledge the important contributions from all those who were kind enough to speak with me about their experiences. Without your amazing insights, my quest to prevent the common cold would not have proven to be successful. Thank you for your willingness to tell your story.

# – CHAPTER SIXTEEN –

# References

The following lists all the references that were made in this book.

[1] Rajnik, M. (2014). Rhinovirus infection, available: Medscape.com
[2] National Health Service (2013). How long do bacteria and viruses this outside the body? Available: Nhs.uk
[3] Tang, J.W., et al. (2013). Airflow Dynamics of Human Jets. Available: Plos.org
[4] Gwaltney, J.M. & Hayden F.G. (1992). Response to psychological stress and susceptibility to the common cold. New England Journal.
[5] Centers for Disease Control (2013). Common Cold and Runny Nose. Available: Cdc.gov
[6] National Library of Medicine (2015). Common Cold. Available: Nih.gov
[7] Centers for Disease Control (2015). Common Colds. Available: Cdc.gov
[8] Fendrick, A.M., et al. (2003). The economic burden of non-influenza-related viral respiratory tract infection United States. Archives of Internal Medicine.
[9] Scientists who study the diseases of ancient man
[10] Holohan, M. (2015). Why do some people never get sick? Link: today.com
[11] Holohan, M. (2015). Why do some people never get sick? Link: today.com
[12] Pauling, L (1976). Vitamin C and the Common Cold. Freeman, SF
[13] Anderson, T.W. (1975). Large-scale trials of vitamin C. Academy of Science
[14] Douglas, R.M. (2007). Vitamin C for preventing and treating the common cold. Available: Nih.gov
[15] Ibid.
[16] Ackerman, J. (2010). How not to fight colds. Available: NYTimes.com
[17] Gwaltney, J.M. & Hayden F.G. (1992). Response to psychological stress and susceptibility to the common cold. New England Journal of Medicine.

[18] Douglas, R.G.J., et al. (1968). Exposure to cold environment and rhinovirus common cold. New England Journal of Medicine.

[19] Douglas, R.G.J., et al. (1968). Exposure to cold environment and rhinovirus common cold. New England Journal of Medicine.

[20] Bock, R. (2008). NIH scientists offer explanation for winter flu season. Available: Nih.gov

[21] Ibid.

[22] Withals, J. (1553). A shorte dictionarie for younge beginners. London

[23] University Health Services (2012). Antibiotics. Available: Berkley.edu

[24] Royal Society of Chemistry (2015). Hydrogen peroxide. Available: Rsc.org

[25] Cameron, D. (2009). Hydrogen peroxide marshals immune system. Available: Harvard.edu

[26] Cameron, D. (2009). Hydrogen peroxide marshals immune system. Available: Harvard.edu

[27] Ibid.

[28] FDA (1983). Hydrogen peroxide: proposed affirmation of GRAS status as a direct human food ingredient with specific limitations. Federal Register 48: 52323-53333

[29] FDA (1988). Oral healthcare drug products for over-the-counter humans uses: tentative final monograph; notice of proposed rulemaking. Federal Register 53: 2436-2461.

[30] Department of Health and Human Services, FDA (2003). Oral healthcare drug production for over-the-counter humans use; antigingivitis/antiplaque drug products; establishment of a monograph. Federal Register 103: 32231-32287

[31] Al-Kerwi, E.A.A., et al. (2005). Mother's milk and hydrogen peroxide. Asia-Pacific Journal for Clinical Nutrition.

[32] Zajic, O. (1999). Disinfection of drinking water with hydrogen peroxide /silver. Fourth international water technology conference IWTC 99.

[33] Tanner, P.A. & Wong, A.Y.S. (1998). Spectrophotometric determination of hydrogen peroxide in rainwater. Analytica Chimica Acta.

[34] Chalishazar, U. & Williams, H. (2007). Back to basics: finding an optimal cerumenolytic (ear wax solvent). British Journal of Nursing.

[35] Senturia B.H. & Doubly J.A. (1947). Treatment of external otitis. III – the use of vehicles and antibiotics in the external auditory canal. In vitro studies. The Laryngoscope 57:633–657.

[36] McCarter, D.F., Courtney, A.U., & Pollart, S.M. (2007). Cerumen impaction. Am Fam Physician, 75(10), 1523-8.

[37] Mercola, J. (2002). Hydrogen peroxide for colds and flu. Available: Mercola.com

[38] Healing Daily (2003). Hydrogen peroxide in the ears. Available. Healingdaily.com

[39] Healing Daily (2003). Hydrogen peroxide in the ears. Available: Healingdaily.com

[40] Mercola, J. (2002). Hydrogen peroxide for colds and flu. Available: Mercola.com

[41] Guarner, F., et al. (2003). Gut flora in health and disease. Available: oranim.ac.il

[42] De Vrese, M., et al. (2006). Probiotic bacteria. Available: researchgate.net

128

[43] Bland, J.S., et al. (1995). A Medical Board-Supplemented Detoxification Program in the Management of Chronic Health Problems. Available: europepmc.org

[44] Denyer, C.V., et al. (1994). Isolation of Antirhinoviral Sesquiterpenes from Ginger (Zingiber officinale). Journal of Natural Products 1994 57 (5), 658-662

[45] Chang, J.S., et al (2013). Fresh ginger has anti-viral activity against human respiratory syncytial virus in human respiratory tract cell lines. Journal of Ethonopharmacology.

[46] Sanchez, A., et al. (1973). Role of sugars in human neutrophilic phagocytosis. American Journal of Clinical Nutrition.

[47] Sanchez, A., et al. (1973). Role of sugars in human neutrophilic phagocytosis. American Journal of Clinical Nutrition.

[48] Rayssiguier, Y., et al. (2006). High fructose consumption combined with low dietary magnesium intake may increase the incidence of the metabolic syndrome by inducing inflammation. Journal of Magnesium Research.

[49] Lombardi, G., et al. (2011). Effect of winter swimming on haematological parameters. Journal of Biochemia Medica.

[50] W.G. Siems , R. Brenke , O. Sommerburg , T. Grune (1999). Improved antioxidative protection in winter swimmers. QJM

[51] Shevchuk, N.A. & Radoja, S. (2007). Possible stimulation of anti-tumor immunity using repeated cold stress: a hypothesis. Infectious Agents and Cancer.

[52] Jacob R.A. & Sotoudeh G. (2002). Vitamin C function and status in chronic disease. Nutr Clin Care.

[53] Hickey, S., et al. (2008). Pharmacokinetics of oral vitamin C. Journal of Nutritional and Environmental Medicine.

[54] Hickey, S., et al. (2008). Pharmacokinetics of oral vitamin C. Journal of Nutritional and Environmental Medicine.

[55] Moyad, M.A., et al. (2008). Effects of a modified yeast supplement on cold/flu symptoms. Urol Nurs.

[56] Ibid.

www.ingramcontent.com/pod-product-compliance
Lightning Source LLC
Chambersburg PA
CBHW070117290526
45789CB00005B/2044